Incomplete penetrance.

assume penetrance 80%

(80% of people ē mutated gene will show that.

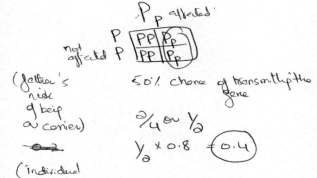

Pp affected

not affected P | PP | Pp |
P | PP | Pp |

(father's risk of being a carrier)

~~0.2~~

50% chance of transmitting the gene

¾ or ½

½ × 0.8 = (0.4)

(individual is not phenotypically affected

→ didn't inherit the mutation

or ē non-penetrant

→ chance he inherited the mutation ½

non penetrant = 1 − penetrance
= 0.2

Chance he transmits the mutation = ½

Child phenotypically affected = 0.8

= ½ × 0.2 × ½ × 0.8 = 0.04

Boards and Beyond:
Biostatistics and Epidemiology Slides

Slides from the Boards and Beyond Website

Jason Ryan, MD, MPH

2019 Edition

| Autosomal Dominant Dominant |

heterozygous individuals will be affected & have 50% chance of transmitting the trait to an offspring. 50% (if the individual heterozygous even ~~heterozygous~~) → 50% chance of transmitting to their child.

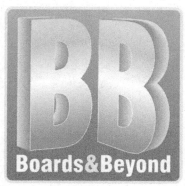

H H
h | Hh | Hh |
h | hh | hh |

H h
h | Hh | hh |
h | Hh | hh |

X linked recessive   (Carrier females, transmit dz to have the males
                       & carrier states to half the females.

	X_D	X
X	X_D X	X x
Y	X_D Y	X Y

& ½/carrier female
X/½

(so 50% of male child can have the dz
50% of female child will be a carrier but no dz)

Table of Contents

Basic Statistics

Jason Ryan, MD, MPH

Statistical Distribution

Random Blood Glucose Healthy Subjects

```
90    115  90    115  90   115  90  115
87    112  87    112  87   112  87  112
101   101 101   101 101   101 101   101
110   92  110   92  110   92   110 92

93    79  93    79   93   79   93  79
      92 100 92 100 92 100 92 100
95    99  95    99   95   99   95  99
88    86  88    86   88   86   88  86
112  102 112  102 112  102 112  102
```

Statistical Distribution
Normal or Gaussian Distribution

No. Subjects (y-axis) vs Blood Glucose Level (x-axis)

Central Tendency

- Center of normal distribution
- Three ways to characterize:
  - Mean: Average of all numbers
  - Median: Middle number of data set when all lined up in order
  - Mode: Most commonly found number

Mean and Mode

- Six blood pressure readings:
  - 90, 80, 80, 100, 110, 120
- Mean = (90+80+80+100+110+120)/6 = 96.7
- Mode is most frequent number = 80

Median

- Odd number of data elements in set
  - 80-90-110
  - Middle number is median = 90
- Even number of data elements
  - 80-90-110-120
  - Halfway between middle pair is median = 100
- Note: Must put data set in order to find median

Central Tendency

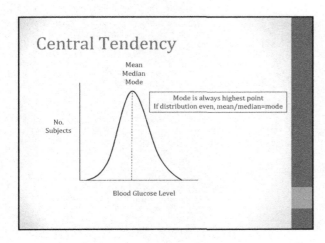

Central Tendency
Negative Skew

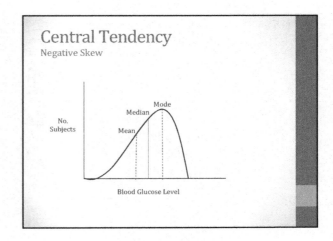

Central Tendency
Positive skew

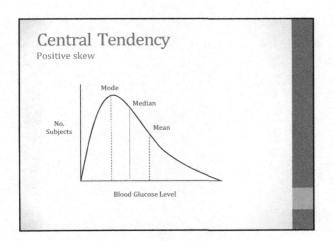

Central Tendency
Key Points

- If distribution is equal, mean=mode=median
- Mode is always at peak
- In skewed data:
  - Mean is always furthest away from mode toward tail
  - Median is between Mean/Mode
- Mode is least likely to be affected by outliers
  - Adding one outlier changes mean, median
  - Only affects mode if it changes most common number
  - Outliers are unlikely to change most common number

Dispersion

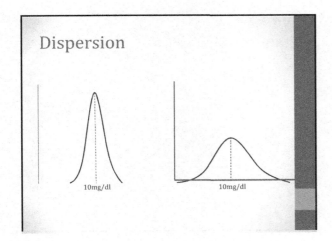

Dispersion Measures

- Standard deviation (SD)
- Variance
- Standard error of the mean (SEM)
- Z-score
- Confidence interval

Standard Deviation

$$\sigma = \sqrt{\frac{\Sigma(x-\bar{x})^2}{n-1}}$$

$x-\bar{x}$ = difference b/w data point and mean

$\Sigma(x-\bar{x})$ = sum of differences

$\Sigma(x-\bar{x})^2$ = sum of differences squared

n = number of samples

Standard Deviation

$$\sigma = \sqrt{\frac{\Sigma(x-\bar{x})^2}{n-1}}$$

Group 1 (mean=10)	Group 2 (mean=10)
9	5
8	6
9	9
10	10
11	12
12	13
10	15
10	14

Standard Deviation

$$\sigma = \sqrt{\frac{\Sigma(x-\bar{x})^c}{n-1}}$$

Group 1 (mean=10)	Difference from mean	Group 2 (mean=10)	Difference from mean
9	-1	5	-5
8	-2	6	-4
9	-1	9	-1
10	0	10	0
11	1	12	2
12	2	13	3
10	0	15	5
10	0	14	4

Standard Deviation

$$\sigma = \sqrt{\frac{\Sigma(x-\bar{x})^2}{n-1}}$$

Group 1 (mean=10)	Difference from mean	Squared	Group 2 (mean=10)	Difference from mean	Squared
9	-1	1	5	-5	25
8	-2	4	6	-4	16
9	-1	1	9	-1	1
10	0	0	10	0	0
11	1	1	12	2	4
12	2	4	13	3	9
10	0	0	15	5	25
10	0	0	14	4	16
		11			96

Standard Deviation

$$\sigma = \sqrt{\frac{\Sigma(x-\bar{x})^2}{n-1}}$$

Group 1 (mean=10)	Difference from mean	Squared	Group 2 (mean=10)	Difference from mean	Squared
9	-1	1	5	-5	25
8	-2	4	6	-4	16
9	-1	1	9	-1	1
10	0	0	10	0	0
11	1	1	12	2	4
12	2	4	13	3	9
10	0	0	15	5	25
10	0	0	14	4	16
		11			96

$$\sigma = \sqrt{\frac{11}{7}} = 1.24$$

$$\sigma = \sqrt{\frac{96}{7}} = 3.7$$

Standard Deviation

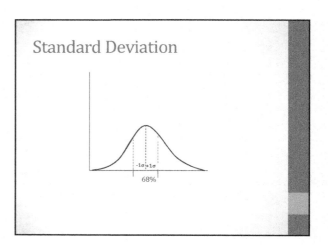

Standard Deviation

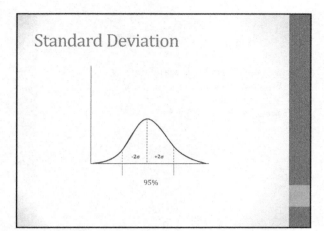

95%

Standard Deviation

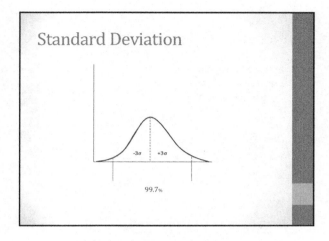

99.7%

Standard Deviation

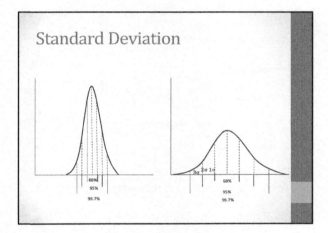

Sample Question

- A test is administered to 200 medical students. The mean score is 80 with a standard deviation of 5. The test scores are normally distributed. How many students scored >90 on the test?
  - 90 is two standard deviations away from mean
  - 2.5% of students score in this range (1/2 of 5%)
  - 2.5% of 200 = 5 students

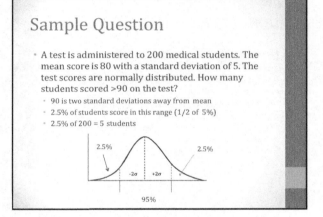

Variance

$$\text{Standard Deviation } \sigma = \sqrt{\frac{\Sigma (x-\bar{x})^2}{n-1}}$$

$$\text{Variance } \sigma^2 = \frac{\Sigma (x-\bar{x})^2}{n}$$

Standard Error of the Mean

- How precisely you know the true population mean
- SD divided by square root of n
- More samples → less SEM (closer to true mean)
- Big σ means big SEM
  - Need lots of samples (n) for small SEM
- Small σ means small SEM
  - Need fewer samples (n) for small SEM

$$\text{SEM} = \frac{\sigma}{\sqrt{n}}$$

Z score

- Z score of 0 is the mean
- Z score of +1 is 1SD above mean
- Z score of -1 is 1SD below mean

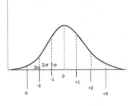

Z score

- Suppose test grade average (mean) = 79
- Standard deviation = 5
- Your grade = 89
- Your Z score = (89-79)/5 = +2

Confidence Intervals

- Mean values often reported with 95% CIs
  - Mean is 120mg/dl +/-5mg/dl
- Range in which 95% of repeated measurements would be expected to fall
- Confidence intervals are for estimating population mean from a sample data set
  - Suppose we take 10 samples of a population of 1M people
  - Mean of 10 samples is X
  - How sure are we the mean of 1M people is also X?
  - Confidence intervals answer this question

Confidence Intervals

- Suppose mean = 10
- SD = 4; n = 16
- SEM = 4/sqrt(16) = 4/4 = 1
- CI = $10 \pm 1.96*(1) = 10 \pm 2$
- 95% of repeated means fall between 8 and 12
  - Upper confidence limit = 12
  - Lower confidence limit = 8

$$\boxed{CI_{95\%} = Mean +/- 1.96*(SEM)}$$

Confidence Intervals

- Don't confuse SD with confidence intervals
- Standard deviation is for a given dataset
  - Suppose we have ten samples
  - These samples have a mean and standard deviation
  - 95% of these samples fall between +/- 2SD
  - This is descriptive characteristic of the sample
- Confidence intervals
  - This does not describe the sample
  - An inferred value of where the true mean lies for *population*

95%

- This value often confusing
- Read carefully: What are they asking for?
- Range in which 95% of measurements in a dataset fall
  - Mean +/- 2SD
- 95% confidence interval of the mean
  - Mean +/- 1.96*SEM

Hypothesis Testing

Jason Ryan, MD, MPH

Hypothesis Testing

- A cardiologist discovers a protein level that may be elevated in myocardial infarction called MIzyme. He wishes to use this to detect heart attacks in the ER. He samples levels of MIzyme among 100 normal subjects and 100 subjects with a myocardial infarction. The mean level in normal subjects is 1mg/dl. The mean level in myocardial infarction patients is 10mg/dl.
- Can this test be used to detect myocardial infarction in the general population?

Hypothesis Testing

- Other way to think about it: Does the mean value of MIzyme in normal subjects truly differ from the mean in myocardial infarction patients?
- Or was the difference in our experiment simply due to chance?
- Depends on several factors:
  - Difference between means normal/MI
  - Scatter of data
  - Number of subjects tested

Hypothesis Testing
Scatter

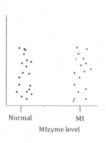

Normal   MI

MIzyme level

Hypothesis Testing
Scatter

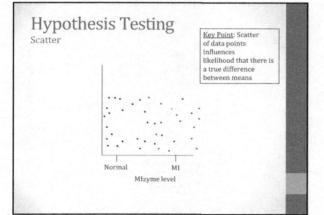

Key Point: Scatter of data points influences likelihood that there is a true difference between means

Normal   MI

MIzyme level

Hypothesis Testing
Number of samples

Key Point: Number of data points influences likelihood that there is a true difference between means

Normal   MI

MIzyme level

Hypothesis Testing

- Hypothesis testing mathematically calculates probabilities (ie. 5% chance, 50% chance) that the two means are truly different and not just different by chance in our experiment
- Math is complex (don't need to know)
- Probabilities by hypothesis testing depends on:
  - Difference between means normal/MI
  - Scatter of data
  - Number of subjects tested

Hypothesis Testing

- Two possibilities of our test of MIzyme
  - #1: MIzyme does NOT distinguish between normal/MI
    - Difference in means was by chance; true means are the same
  - #2: MIzyme DOES distinguish between normal/MI
    - Difference in means is real
- Null hypothesis (H_0) = #1
- Alternative hypothesis (H_1) = #2

Hypothesis Testing

- In reality, either H_0 or H_1 is correct
- In our experiment, either H_0 or H_1 will be deemed correct
- Hypothesis testing determines likelihood our experiment matches with reality

Hypothesis Testing

- Four possible outcomes of our experiment:
  - #1: There is a difference in reality and our experiment detects it. This means the alternative hypothesis (H_1) is found true by our study.
  - #2: There is no difference in reality and our experiment also finds no difference. This means the null hypothesis (H_0) is found true by our study.
  - #3: There is no difference in reality but our study finds a difference. This is an error! Type 1 (α) error.
  - #4: There is a difference in reality but our study misses it. This is also an error! Type 2 (β) error.

Hypothesis Testing

- Each of the four outcomes has a probability of being correct based on:
  - Difference between means normal/MI
  - Scatter of data
  - Number of subjects tested

Hypothesis Testing

Reality

Experiment	H_1	H_0
H_1	Power	α
H_0	β	H_0 Correct

Power = Chance of detecting difference
α = Chance of seeing difference that is not real
β = chance of missing a difference that is really there
Power = 1- β

Power

- Chance of finding a difference when one exists
- Or chance of rejecting no difference (because there really is one)
  - Also called rejecting the null hypothesis (H_0)
- Power is increased when:
  - Increased sample size
  - Large difference of means
  - Less scatter of data (more precise measurements)

Power

- Maximize power to detect a true difference
- In study design, you have little/no control over:
  - Scatter of data
  - Difference between means
- You DO have control over
  - Number of subjects
- Number of subjects chosen to give a high power
- This is called a power calculation

Statistical Errors

- Type 1 (α) error
  - False positive
  - Finding a difference/effect when there is none in reality
  - Rejecting null hypothesis (H_0) when you should not have
  - Example: Researchers conclude a drug benefits patients but it dose not
  - Null hypothesis generally not rejected unless $\alpha < 0.05$
- Similar (but different) from p value
  - p value calculated by comparison
  - α set by study design

Statistical Errors

- Type 2 (β) error
  - False negative
  - Finding no difference/effect when there is one in reality
  - Accepting null hypothesis (H_0) when you should not have
  - Example: Researchers conclude a drug does not benefit patients but a later study finds that it does
  - Can get type 2 error if too few patients

Tests of Significance

Jason Ryan, MD, MPH

Comparing Groups

- Many clinical studies compare group means
- Often find differences between groups
  - Different mean ages
  - Different mean blood levels, etc.
- Need to compare differences to determine the

  - Are the differences "statistically significant?"

Comparing Groups

Little scatter of data in groups
Groups far apart relative to scatter

Group 1   Group 2
Test Result

Comparing Groups

Lots of scatter of data in groups
Groups not far apart relative to scatter

Group 1   Group 2
Test Result

Key Point

- Scatter of data points relative to difference in means influences likelihood that difference between means is due to chance
- This is how differences between means are tested to determine likelihood that they are different due to chance
- Don't need to know the math
- Just understand principle

Comparing Groups

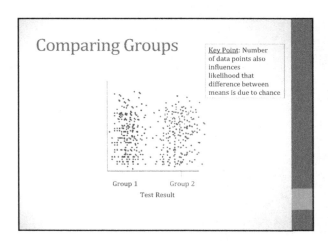

Key Point: Number of data points also influences likelihood that difference between means is due to chance

Group 1   Group 2
Test Result

Comparing Groups

- Three key tests
  - t-test
  - ANOVA
  - Chi-square
- Determine likelihood difference between means is due to chance
- Likelihood of difference due to chance based on
  - Scatter of data points
  - How far apart the means are from each other
  - Number of data points

Data Types

- Quantitative variables:
  - 1, 2, 3, 4
- Categorical variables:
  - High, medium, low
  - Positive, negative
  - Yes, No
- Quantitative variables often reported as number
  - Mean age was 62 years old
- Categorical variables often report as percentages
  - 40% of patients take drug A
  - 20% of patients are heavy exercisers

T-test

- Compares two MEAN quantitative values
- Yields a p-value
- p value is chance that the null hypothesis is correct
  - No difference between means
- If $p<0.05$ we usually reject the null hypothesis and state that the difference in means is "statistically significant"

T-test

- A researcher studies plasma levels of sodium in patients with SIADH and normal patients. The mean value in SIADH patients is 128mg/dl with a standard deviation of 2. The mean value in normal patients is 136mg/dl with a standard deviation of 3. Is this difference significant?
- Common questions:
  - Which test to compare the means? (t-test)
  - What p-value indicates significance? (<0.05)

T-test

- A researcher studies plasma levels of sodium in patients with SIADH and normal patients. The mean value in SIADH patients is 128mg/dl with a standard deviation of 2. The mean value in normal patients is 136mg/dl with a standard deviation of 3. Is this difference significant?
- If the p value is high (non-significant) why might that be the case?
  - Need more patients
  - Increase sample size → increase power to detect differences

ANOVA

- Analysis of variance
- Used to compare more than two quantitative means
- Consider:
  - Plasma level of creatinine determined in non-pregnant, pregnant, and post-partum women
  - Three means determined
  - Cannot use t-test (two means only)
  - Use ANOVA
- Yields a p-value like t-tests

Chi-square

- Compares two or more categorical variables
- Must use this test if results are not hard numbers
- When asked to choose statistical test for a dataset always ask yourself whether data is quantitative or categorical
- Beware of percentages – often categorical data

Confidence Intervals

- Sixteen normal subjects have their blood glucose level sampled. The mean blood glucose level is 90mg/dl with a standard deviation of 4md/dl. What is the likelihood that the mean glucose level of another ten subjects would also be 90mg/dl?
- How confident are we in the number 90mg/dl?

Confidence Intervals

- In scientific literature, means are reported with a confidence interval
  - Study subjects: Mean glucose was 90 +/- 4
- Authors believe that if the study subjects were re-sampled, the mean result would fall between 86 and 94 for 95% of re-samples
- For 5% of re-samples, the result would fall outside of 86 to 94

Confidence Intervals

- To calculate a confidence interval you need 2 things
  - Standard deviation (σ)
  - Number of subjects tested to find mean value (n)

$$\text{Confidence Interval} = +/- Z * \frac{\sigma}{\sqrt{n}}$$

Z = 1.96 for 95% CI
Z = 2.58 for 99% CI

Confidence Interval

- Sixteen normal subjects have their blood glucose level sampled. The mean blood glucose level is 90mg/dl with a standard deviation of 4md/dl. What is the likelihood that the mean glucose level of another sixteen subjects would also be 90mg/dl?

$$\text{Confidence Interval} = \pm Z * \frac{\sigma}{\sqrt{n}} = \pm 1.96 * \frac{4}{\sqrt{16}} = \pm 1.96 \approx 2$$

95% chance that next 16 samples would fall between 88 and 92mg/dl

Confidence Interval

- Don't confuse with standard deviation
- Mean +/- 2SD
  - 95% of samples fall in this range
- Mean +/- CI
  - 95% chance that repeated measurement of mean in this range
- If you see 95% in a question stem
  - Read carefully: What are they asking for?
  - Range of 95% of samples?
  - 95% confidence interval of mean?

Odds and Risk Ratios

- Some studies report odds or risk ratios with CIs
- If range includes 1.0 then exposure/risk factor does not significantly impact disease/outcome
- Example:
  - Risk of lung cancer among chemical workers studied
  - Risk ratio = 1.4 +/- 0.5
  - Confidence interval includes 1.0
  - Chemical work not significantly associated with lung cancer
  - (Formal statement: Null hypothesis not rejected)

Confidence Intervals
Group Comparisons

- Many studies report differences between groups
- Can average differences and calculate CIs
- If includes zero, no statistically significant difference
- Example:
  - Mean difference between two groups is 1.0 +/- 3.0
  - Includes zero
  - No significant difference between groups
  - Similar to p>0.05
  - (Formal statement: Null hypothesis not rejected)

Confidence Intervals
Group Comparisons

- Some studies report group means with CIs
- If ranges overlap, no statistically significant difference
- Group 1 mean: 10 +/- 5; Group 2 mean: 8 +/-4
  - Confidence intervals overlap
  - No significant difference between means
  - Similar to p>0.05 for comparison of means
- Group 1 mean: 10 +/- 5; Group 2 mean: 30 +/-4
  - Confidence intervals do not overlap
  - Significant difference between means
  - Similar to p<0.05 for comparison of means

Correlations

Jason Ryan, MD, MPH

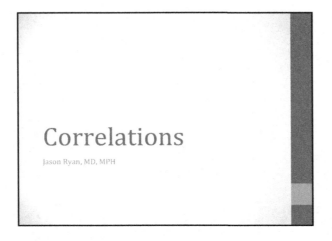

Correlation Coefficient
Pearson Coefficient

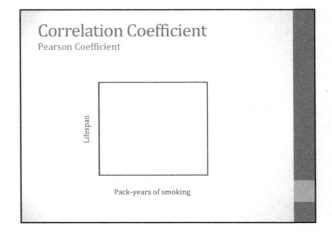

Lifespan

Pack-years of smoking

Correlation Coefficient
Pearson Coefficient

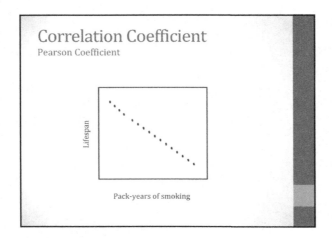

Lifespan

Pack-years of smoking

Correlation Coefficient
Pearson Coefficient

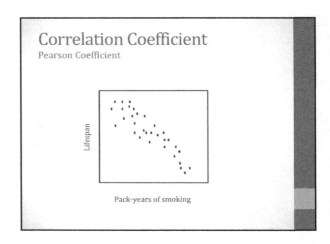

Lifespan

Pack-years of smoking

Correlation Coefficient
Pearson Coefficient

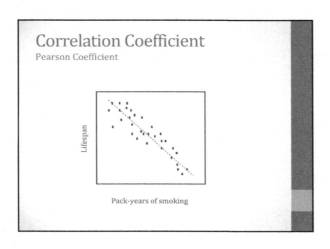

Lifespan

Pack-years of smoking

Correlation Coefficient
Pearson Coefficient

- Measure of linear correlation between two variables
- Represents strength of association of two variables
- Number from -1 to +1
- Closer to 1, stronger the relationship
- (-) number means inverse relationship
  - More smoking, less lifespan
- (+) number means positive relationship
  - More smoking, more lifespan
- 0 means no relationship

Correlation Coefficient
Pearson Coefficient

Strength of Relationship

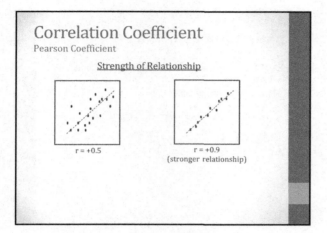

r = +0.5

r = +0.9
(stronger relationship)

Correlation Coefficient
Pearson Coefficient

Direction of Relationship

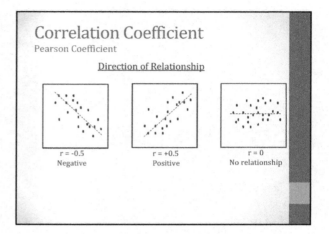

r = -0.5
Negative

r = +0.5
Positive

r = 0
No relationship

Correlation Coefficient
Pearson Coefficient

- Studies will report relationships with CC
- Example:
  - Study of pneumonia patients
  - WBC on admission evaluated for relationship LOS
  - r = +0.5
  - Higher WBC → Higher LOS
- Sometimes a p value is also reported
  - P<0.05 indicates significant correlation
  - p>0.05 indicates no significant correlation

Coefficient of Determination
r^2

- Sometimes r^2 reported instead of r
- Always positive
- Indicates % of variation in y explained by x

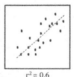
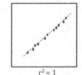

$r^2 = 0.6$
(60% variation y explained by x)

$r^2 = 1$
(100% variation y explained by x)

Study Designs

Jason Ryan, MD, MPH

Epidemiology Studies

- Goal: Determine if exposure/risk factor associated with disease
- Many real world examples
  - Hypertension → stroke
  - Smoking → lung cancer
  - Toxic waste → leukemia

Types of Studies

Determine association of exposure/risk with disease

- Cross-sectional study
- Case-control study
- Cohort study (prospective/retrospective)

Cross-sectional Study

- Patients studied based on being part of a group
  - New Yorkers
  - Women
  - Tall people
- Frequency of disease and risk factors identified
  - How many have lung cancer?
  - How many smoke?
- Snapshot in time
  - Patients not followed for months/years

Cross-sectional Study

- Main outcome of this study is **prevalence**
  - 50% of New Yorkers smoke
  - 25% of New Yorkers have lung cancer
- May have more than one group
  - 50% men have lung cancer, 25% of women have lung cancer
  - But groups not followed over time (i.e. years)
- Can't determine:
  - How much smoking increases risk of lung cancer (RR)
  - Odds of getting lung cancer in smokers vs. non-smokers (OR)

Cross-sectional Study

- New Yorkers were surveyed to determine whether they smoke and whether they have morning cough. The study found a smoking prevalence of 50%. Among responders, 25% reported morning cough.
- Note the absence of a time period
  - Patients not followed for 1-year, etc.
- Likely questions:
  - Type of study? (cross-sectional)
  - What can be determined? (prevalence of disease)

Cross-sectional Study

- Using a national US database, rates of lung cancer were determined among New Yorkers, Texans, and Californians. Lung cancer prevalence was 25% in New York, 30% in Texas, and 20% in California. The researchers concluded that living in Texas is associated with higher rates of lung cancer.
- Key points:
  - Presence of different groups could make you think of other study types
  - However, note lack of time frame
  - Study is just a fancy description of disease prevalence

Cross-sectional Study

- Researchers discover a gene that they believe leads to development of diabetes. A sample of 1000 patients is randomly selected. All patients are screened for the gene. Presence or absence of diabetes is determined from a patient questionnaire. It is determined that the gene is strongly associated with diabetes.
- Key points:
  - Note lack of time frame
  - Patients not selected by disease or exposure (random)
  - Just a snapshot in time

Case Series

- Purely descriptive study (similar to cross-sectional)
- Often used in new diseases with unclear cause
- Multiple cases of a condition combined/analyzed
  - Patient demographics (age, gender)
  - Symptoms
- Done to look for clues about etiology/course
- No control group

Cohort Study

- Compares group with exposure to group without
- Did exposure change likelihood of disease?
- Prospective
  - Monitor groups over time
- Retrospective
  - Look back in time at groups

Cohort Study

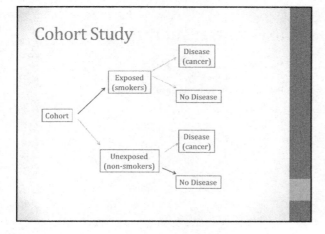

Cohort Study

- Main outcome measure is relative risk (RR)
  - How much does exposure increase risk of disease
- Patients identified by **risk factor** (i.e. smoking or non)
  - Different from case-control (by *disease*)
- Example results
  - 50% smokers get lung cancer within 5 years
  - 10% non-smokers get lung cancer within 5 years
  - RR = 50/10 = 5
  - Smokers 5 times more likely to get lung cancer

Cohort Study

- A group of 100 New Yorkers who smoke were identified based on a screening questionnaire at a local hospital. These patients were compared to another group that reported no smoking. Both groups received follow-up surveys asking about development of lung cancer annually for the next 3 years. The prevalence of lung cancer was 25% among smokers and 5% among non-smokers.
- Likely questions:
  - Type of study? (*prospective* cohort)
  - What can be determined? (relative risk)

Cohort Study

- A group of 100 New Yorkers who smoke were identified based on a screening questionnaire at a local hospital. These patients were compared to another group that reported no smoking. Hospital records were analyzed going back 5 years for all patients. The prevalence of lung cancer was 25% among smokers and 5% among non-smokers.
- Likely questions:
  - Type of study? (*retrospective* cohort)
  - What can be determined? (relative risk)

Cohort Study

- Problem: Does not work with rare diseases
- Imagine:
  - 100 smokers, 100 non-smokers
  - Followed over 1 year
  - Zero cases of lung cancer both groups
- In rare diseases need LOTS of patients for LONG time
- Easier to find **cases** of lung cancer first then compare to cases without lung cancer

Case-control study

- Compares group with disease to group without
- Looks for exposure or risk factors
- Opposite of cohort study
- Better for rare diseases

Case-Control Study

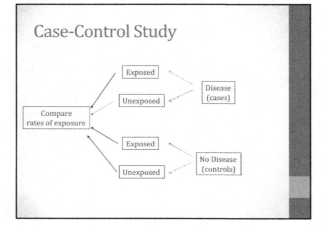

Case-control study

- Main outcome measure is odds ratio
  - Odds of disease exposed/odds of disease unexposed
- Patients identified by **disease** or no disease

Case-control study

- A group of 100 New Yorkers with lung cancer were identified based on a screening questionnaire at a local hospital. These patients were compared to another group that reported no lung cancer. Both groups were questioned about smoking within the past 10 years. The prevalence of smoking was 25% among lung cancer patients and 5% among non-lung cancer patients.
- Likely questions:
  - Type of study? (case-control)
  - What can be determined? (odds ratio)

Matching

- Selection of control group (matching) key to getting good study results
- Want patients as close to disease patients as possible (except for disease)
- Matching reduces confounding
- Want all potential confounders balanced between cases and controls

Randomized Trials

- Don't confuse with case-control
- Patients identified by disease like case-control
- Exposure determined **randomly**

Case-control vs. Cohort

Case Control	Cohort
Patients by disease	Patients by exposure
Odds ratio	Relative Risk

How to Identify Study Types?

- #1: How were patients identified?
  - Cross-sectional: By location/group (i.e. New Yorkers)
  - Cohort: By exposure/risk factors (i.e. Smokers)
  - Case-control: By disease (i.e. Lung cancer)

How to Identify Study Types?

- #2: Time period of the study
  - Cross-sectional: No time period (i.e. snapshot)
  - Retrospective: Look backward for disease/exposure
  - Prospective: Follow forward in time for disease/exposure

How to Identify Study Types?

- #3: What numbers are determined from study?
  - Cross-sectional: Prevalence of disease (possibly by group)
  - Cohort: Relative risk (RR)
  - Case-control: Odds ratio (OR)

Risk Quantification

Jason Ryan, MD, MPH

Why Risk is Important

- Understanding of disease causes comes from estimating risk
  - Smoking increases risk of lung cancer
  - Exercise decreases risk of heart attacks
- We know these things from quantifying risk
  - Smoking increases risk of lung cancer X percent
  - Exercise decreases risk of heart attacks Y percent

Data for Risk Estimation

- Obtained by studying:
  - Presence/absence of risk factor/exposure
  - In people with and without disease
- Cohort study
- Case-control study

The 2 x 2 Table

		Disease +	Disease -
Exposure	+	A	B
	-	C	D

Uses of the 2x2 Table

- Can calculate many things:
  - Risk of disease
  - Risk ratio
  - Odds ratio
  - Attributable risk
  - Number needed to harm

Risk of Disease

- Risk in exposed group = A/(A+B)
- Risk in unexposed group = C/(C+D)

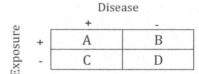

		Disease +	Disease -
Exposure	+	A	B
	-	C	D

Risk Ratio

- Risk of disease with exposure vs non-exposure
  - RR = 5
    - Smokers 5x more likely to get lung cancer than nonsmokers
- Usually from cohort study
- Ranges from zero to infinity
  - RR = 1 → No increased risk from exposure
  - RR > 1 → Exposure increases risk
  - RR < 1 → Exposure decreases risk

Risk Ratio

Disease

Exposure	+	-
+	A	B
-	C	D

$$RR = \frac{A/(A+B)}{C/(C+D)}$$

Risk Ratio

- Example #1:
  - 10% smokers get lung cancer
  - 10% nonsmokers get lung cancer
  - RR = 1

Risk Ratio

- Example #2:
  - 50% smokers get lung cancer
  - 10% nonsmokers get lung cancer
  - RR = 5

Risk Ratio

- Example #3:
  - 10% smokers get lung cancer
  - 50% nonsmokers get lung cancer
  - RR = 0.2
  - Smoking protective!

Risk Ratio

- A group of 1000 college students is evaluated over ten years. Two hundred are smokers and 800 are non-smokers. Over the 10 year study period, 50 smokers get lung cancer compared with 10 non-smokers.

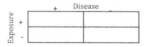

$$RR = \frac{A/(A+B)}{C/(C+D)} = \underline{\hspace{2cm}}$$

Odds Ratio

- Usually from case control study
- Odds of exposure-disease/odds exposure-no-disease
- Ranges from zero to infinity
  - OR = 1 → Exposure equal among disease/no-disease
  - OR > 1 → Exposure increased among disease/no-disease
  - OR < 1 → Exposure decreased among disease/no-disease

Odds Ratio

Disease

Exposure		+	-
	+	A	B
	-	C	D

$$OR = \frac{A/C}{B/D} = \frac{A*D}{B*C}$$

Odds Ratio

- Example #1:
  - 10x lung cancer patients smoke vs. non-smokers
  - 10x non-lung cancer patients smoke vs. non-smokers
  - OR = 1

Odds Ratio

- Example #2:
  - 50x lung cancer patients smoke vs. non-smokers
  - 10x non-lung cancer patients smoke vs. non-smokers
  - OR = 5

Odds Ratio

- Example #3:
  - 10x lung cancer patients smoke vs. non-smokers
  - 50x non-lung cancer patients smoke vs. non-smokers
  - OR = 0.2

Risk vs. Odds Ratio

- Risk ratio is the preferred metric
  - Easy to understand
  - Tells you how much exposure increase risk
- Why not calculate it in all studies?
  - Not valid in case-control studies
  - RR is different depending on number cases you choose

Risk vs. Odds Ratio

Suppose we find 100 cases and 200 controls
RR = $\frac{50/100}{50/200}$ = 2.0

Lung Cancer

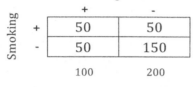

		+	-
Smoking	+	50	50
	-	50	150
		100	200

Risk vs. Odds Ratio

Now suppose we find 200 cases and 200 controls
RR = $\frac{100/150}{100/250}$ = 1.6

Lung Cancer

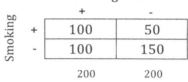

		+	-
Smoking	+	100	50
	-	100	150
		200	200

Risk vs. Odds Ratio

OR does not change with case number

	+	-
+	50	50
-	50	150
	100	200

	+	-
+	100	50
-	100	150
	200	200

OR = $\frac{50/50}{50/150}$ = 3.0

OR = $\frac{100/100}{50/150}$ = 3.0

Risk vs. Odds Ratio

- Risk ratio is dependent on number of cases/controls
- Invalid to use risk ratio in case-control
- Must use odds ratio instead

Rare Disease Assumption

$$OR = \frac{A/C}{B/D} = \frac{A*D}{B*C}$$

$$RR = \frac{A/(A+B)}{C/(C+D)} = \frac{A/B}{C/D} = \frac{A*D}{B*C}$$

OR = RR
When B>>A and D>>C

Rare Disease Assumption

Disease

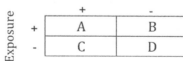

		+	-
Exposure	+	A	B
	-	C	D

OR = RR
When B>>A and D>>C

Rare Disease Assumption

- OR = RR
- Most exposed/unexposed have no disease (-)
- Few disease (+) among exposed/unexposed

Rare Disease Assumption

- Allows use of a case-control study to determine RR
- Commonly accepted number is prevalence <10%
- Case-control studies easy/cheap
  - But odds ratio is weak association
- Classic question:
  - Description of case-control study
  - RR reported
  - Is this valid?
  - Answer: Only if disease is rare

Attributable Risk

- Suppose 1% chance lung cancer in non-smokers
- Suppose 21% chance in smokers
- Attributable risk = 20%
- Added risk due to exposure to smoking

Attributable Risk

Disease

	+	-
+	A	B
-	C	D

Exposure

$$AR = A/(A+B) - C/(C+D)$$

Attributable Risk Percentage

- (risk exposed – risk unexposed)/risk exposed
- Represents % disease explained by risk factor
  - Supposed ARP for smoking and lung cancer 80%
  - Indicates 80% of lung cancers explained by smoking
- Can be calculated directly from RR

$$ARP = \frac{RR - 1}{RR}$$

Number Need to Harm

- Number of patients on average needed to be exposed for one episode of disease on average to occur
- Example: Average number of people who need to smoke for one case of lung cancer to develop
- If attributable risk to smoking is 20%, then NNH is 1/0.2 = 5

$$NNH = \frac{1}{AR}$$

Sensitivity and Specificity

Jason Ryan, MD, MPH

Incidence and Prevalence

- Suppose 1,000 new cases diabetes per year
  - This is the **incidence** of diabetes
- Suppose 100,000 cases of diabetes at one point in time
  - This is the **prevalence** of diabetes for population

Incidence and Prevalence

- Incidence rate = new cases / population at risk
  - Determined for a period of time (e.g. one year)
  - Population at risk = total pop – people with disease
  - 40,000 people
  - 10,000 with disease
  - 1,000 new cases per year
  - Incidence rate = 1,000 / (40k-10k) = 1,000 cases/30,000
- Prevalence rate = number of cases / population at risk
  - Entire population at risk

Incidence and Prevalence

- For chronic diseases
  - Prevalence >> incidence
- For rapidly fatal diseases
  - Incidence ~ prevalence
- New primary prevention programs
  - Both incidence and prevalence fall
- New drugs that improve survival
  - Incidence unchanged
  - Prevalence increases

Diagnostic Tests

Blood Glucose Levels

Normal Subjects			Diabetics		
90	115	90	140	115	140
87	112	87	132	112	132
101	101	101	110	101	110
110	92	110	105	176	105
105	85	105	127	180	127
93	79	93	170	199	170
92	100	92	140	100	140
95	99	95	160	143	160
88	86	88	112	168	112
112	102	112	160	102	160

Diagnostic Tests

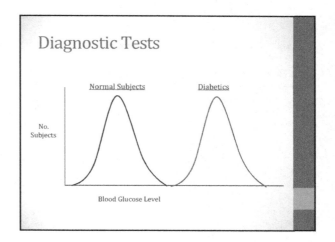

Diagnostic Tests

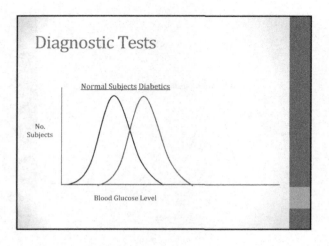

Diagnostic Tests

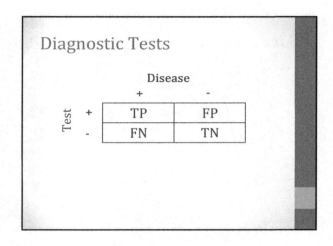

Sensitivity

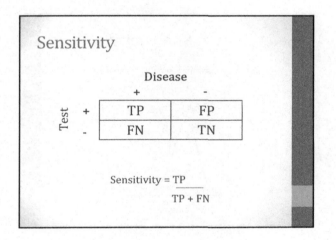

Sensitivity

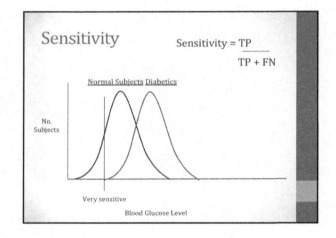

Sensitivity

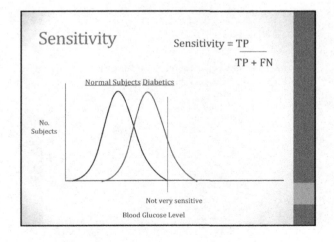

Specificity

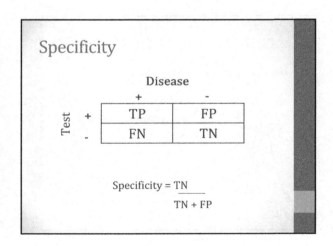

Specificity

$$\text{Specificity} = \frac{TN}{TN + FP}$$

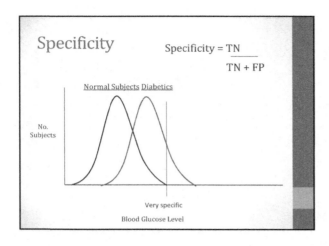

Specificity

$$\text{Specificity} = \frac{TN}{TN + FP}$$

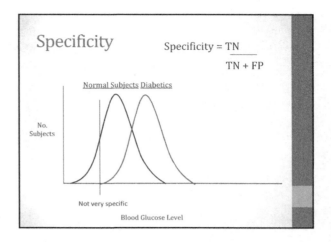

Sample Question

- The results below are obtained from a study of test X on patients with and without disease A. What is the sensitivity of test X?

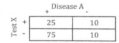

		Disease A	
		+	-
Test X	+	25	10
	-	75	10

Sensitivity & Specificity

- Midpoint cutoff maximizes sensitivity/specificity

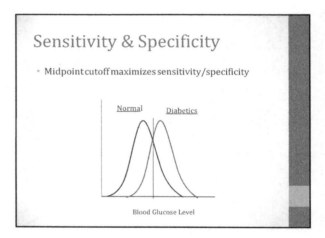

Sensitivity & Specificity

- Degree of overlap limits max combined sens/spec

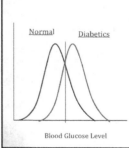 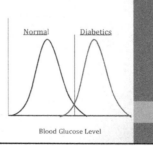

Key Point

- High sensitivity = good at ruling OUT disease
- High specificity = good at ruling IN disease

Key Point

- Sensitivity/Specificity are characteristics of the test
- Remain constant for any prevalence of disease

Sensitivity/Specificity

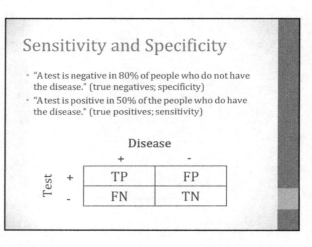

Sensitivity/Specificity

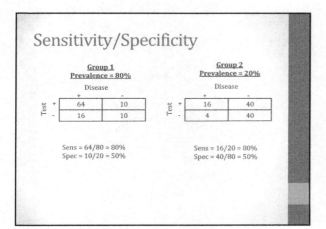

Sensitivity and Specificity

- "A test is negative in 80% of people who do not have the disease." (true negatives; specificity)
- "A test is positive in 50% of the people who do have the disease." (true positives; sensitivity)

		Disease	
		+	-
Test	+	TP	FP
	-	FN	TN

Sensitivity and Specificity

- Use sensitive tests when you don't want to miss cases
  - Captures many true positives (at cost of false positives)
  - Screening of large populations
  - Severe diseases
- Use specific tests after sensitive tests
  - Confirmatory tests
- Specific tests often more costly/cumbersome
  - Performed only if screening (sensitive) test positive

Positive and Negative Predictive Value

Jason Ryan, MD, MPH

Implications of Test Results

- I have a positive result. What is likelihood I have disease?
- I have a negative result. What is likelihood I don't have disease?
- Sensitivity/Specificity do not answer these questions
- For this we need:
  - Positive predictive value
  - Negative predictive value

Positive Predictive Value

		Disease +	Disease -
Test	+	TP	FP
	-	FN	TN

$$PPV = \frac{TP}{TP + FP}$$

Negative Predictive Value

		Disease +	Disease -
Test	+	TP	FP
	-	FN	TN

$$NPV = \frac{TN}{TN + FN}$$

Sample Question

- A test has a sensitivity of 80% and a specificity of 50%. The test is used in a population where disease prevalence is 40%. What is the positive predictive value?

		Disease A +	-
Test X	+	32	30
	-	8	30

40 patients   60 patients   100 patients

$$PPV = \frac{TP}{TP + FP} = \frac{32}{62} = 52\%$$

Key Point

- Unlike sensitivity/specificity, PPV/NPV are highly dependent on the prevalence of disease

Positive Predictive Value

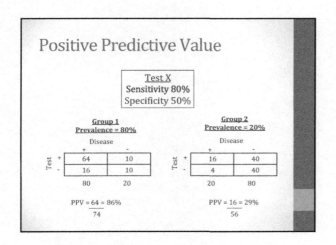

Test X
Sensitivity 80%
Specificity 50%

Group 1
Prevalence = 80%

Test	Disease +	Disease -
+	64	10
-	16	10
	80	20

$PPV = \dfrac{64}{74} = 86\%$

Group 2
Prevalence = 20%

Test	Disease +	Disease -
+	16	40
-	4	40
	20	80

$PPV = \dfrac{16}{56} = 29\%$

Negative Predictive Value

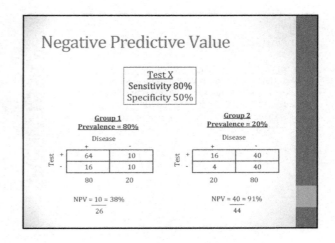

Test X
Sensitivity 80%
Specificity 50%

Group 1
Prevalence = 80%

Test	Disease +	Disease -
+	64	10
-	16	10
	80	20

$NPV = \dfrac{10}{26} = 38\%$

Group 2
Prevalence = 20%

Test	Disease +	Disease -
+	16	40
-	4	40
	20	80

$NPV = \dfrac{40}{44} = 91\%$

Key Point

- PPV is higher when prevalence is higher
- NPV is high when prevalence is lower

Cutoff Point and PPV/NPV

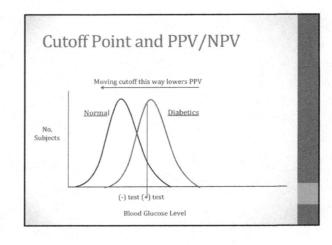

Moving cutoff this way lowers PPV

No. Subjects

Normal   Diabetics

(-) test (+) test

Blood Glucose Level

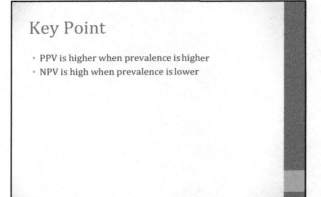

$$PPV = \frac{TP}{TP + FP}$$

	Cutoff A	Cutoff B
TP	10	15
FP	5	10
PPV	10/15 = 66%	15/25 = 60%

Normal Subjects   Diabetics

No. Subjects

B   A

Blood Glucose Level

Cutoff Point and PPV/NPV

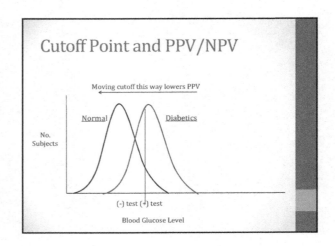

Moving cutoff this way lowers PPV

No. Subjects

Normal   Diabetics

(-) test (+) test

Blood Glucose Level

Sample Question

- The American Diabetes Association proposes lowering the cutoff value for the fasting glucose level that indicates diabetes. How will this change effect sensitivity, specificity, PPV, and NPV?
  - Sensitivity: Increase
  - Specificity: Decrease
  - PPV: Decrease
  - NPV: Increase

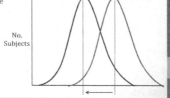

Diagnostic Tests

Jason Ryan, MD, MPH

Diagnostic Tests
Special Topics

- Accuracy/Precision
- ROC Curves
- Likelihood ratios

Accuracy vs. Precision

- Accuracy (validity) is how closely data matches reality
- Precision (reliability) is how closely repeated measurements match each other
- Can have accuracy without precision (or vice versa)

Accuracy and Precision

- More precise tests have smaller standard deviations
- Less precise tests have larger standard deviations

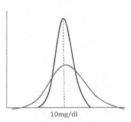

10mg/dl

Accuracy vs. Precision

- Random measurement errors: reduce precision of test
  - Imagine some measurements okay, others bad (random error)
  - Accuracy may be maintained but lots of data scatter
- Systemic errors reduce accuracy
  - Imagine every BP measurement off by 10mmHg due to wrong cuff size (systemic error in data set)
  - Precision okay but accuracy is off

ROC Curves
Receiver Operating Characteristic

- Tests have different sensitivity/specificity depending on the cutoff value chosen
- Which cutoff value maximizes sensitivity/specificity?
- ROC curves answer this question

ROC Curve

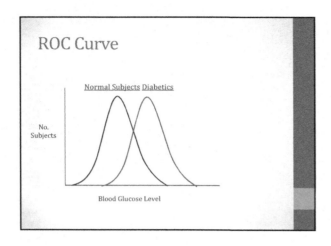

ROC Curves

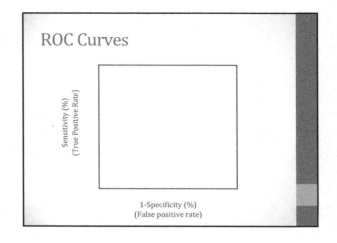

ROC Curves

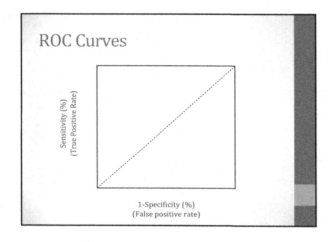

ROC Curves

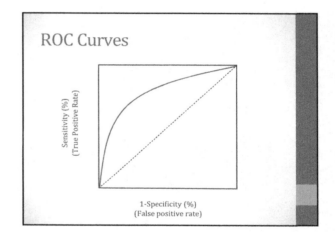

ROC Curves

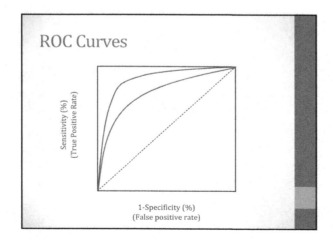

ROC Curves

- Straight line from bottom left to top right is a bad test
- Closer curve is to right angle, better the test

ROC Curves

- Point closest to top left corner is best cutoff to maximize sensitivity/specificity

(graph: y-axis: Sensitivity (%) (True Positive Rate))

Area Under Curve

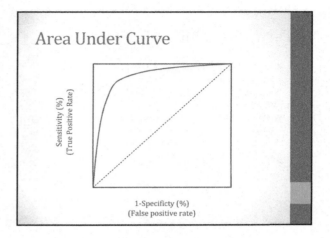

(graph: y-axis: Sensitivity (%) (True Positive Rate); x-axis: 1-Specificty (%) (False positive rate))

ROC: Area Under Curve

- Useless test has 0.5 (50%) area under curve
- Perfect test has 1.0 (100%) area under curve
- More area under curve = better test
  - More ability to discriminate individuals with disease from those without

Likelihood Ratios

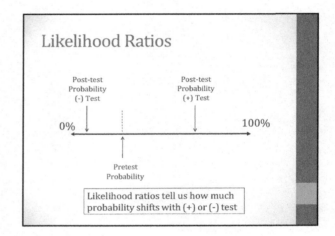

Post-test Probability (-) Test

Post-test Probability (+) Test

0%   100%

Pretest Probability

Likelihood ratios tell us how much probability shifts with (+) or (-) test

Likelihood Ratios

$$LR^+ = \frac{Sensitivity}{1 - Specificity}$$

$$LR^- = \frac{1 - Sensitivity}{Specificity}$$

These are characteristics of test like sensitivity/specificity
Do not vary with prevalence of disease
Need to know pre-test probability to use LRs

Likelihood Ratios

LR	Interpretation
>10	Large increase probability
1	No change in probability
<0.1	Large decrease in probability

Term: "Likelihood"

- What is likelihood of disease in a person with (+) test?
  - Positive predictive value
- What is likelihood of disease in a person with (-) test?
  - Negative predictive value
- What is the positive likelihood ratio?
  - Calculated from sensitivity/specificity
- What is the negative likelihood ratio?
  - Calculated from sensitivity/specificity

Bias

Jason Ryan, MD, MPH

Bias

- Bias = systematic error in a study
- Suppose a study found exposure to chemical X increased headaches by 40% vs. non-exposure
- How could this be wrong?
  - Selected/sampled groups incorrectly
  - Assessed presence/absence of headache incorrectly

Selection Bias

- Groups differ in ways other than exposure
- Example: Volunteers are exposed and compared with general population that is not exposed
  - Volunteers may differ in many ways from general population
- Example: Workers exposed compared with general population
  - Workers may differ in many ways
- Usually used as a general term
- If groups differ specifically by one factor (e.g., smoking) that affects outcome → confounding/effect modification

Attrition Bias
Type of selection bias

- Problem in prospective studies
- Patients **lost to follow-up** unequally between groups
- Patients who do not follow-up excluded from analysis
  - By not following up, patients *selecting* out of trial
  - Or by following up, patients *selecting* to be in trial
- Suppose 100 smokers lost to follow-up due to death
- Study may show smoking less harmful than reality

Sampling Bias
Type of selection bias

- Patient's in trial **not representative** of actual practice
- Results non generalizable to clinical practice
- Average age many heart failure trials = 65
- Average age actual heart failure patients = 80+
- Trial results may not apply

Berkson's Bias
Type of selection bias

- Selection bias when hospitalized patients chosen as treatment or control arm
- May have more severe symptoms
- May have better access to care
- Alters results of study

Confounding Bias

- Unmeasured factor confounds study results
- Example:
  - Alcoholics appear to get more lung cancer than non-alcoholics
  - Smoking much more prevalent among alcoholics
  - Smoking is true cause of more cancer
  - Smoking is a confounder of results

Stratified Analysis
Eliminates Confounding Bias

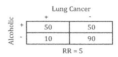

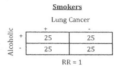
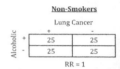

Controlling for Confounders

- Randomization
  - Ensures equal variables in both arms
- Matching
  - Case-control studies
  - Careful selection of control subjects
  - Goal is to match case subjects as closely as possible
  - Choose patients with same age, gender, etc.

Hawthorne Effect

- Study patients improve because they are being studied
- Patients or providers change behavior based on being studied
- Common in studies of behavioral patterns
- Examples:
  - Physicians know their patients are being surveyed about vaccination status → physicians vaccinate more often
  - Patients know they are being studied for exercise capacity → patients exercise more often

Pygmalion Effect
Observer-expectancy effect

- Researcher believes in efficacy of treatment
- Influences outcome of study
- Example:
  - The creator of a new surgical device uses it on his own patients as part of a clinical trial

Pygmalion vs. Hawthorne

- Pygmalion effect
  - Provider believes in treatment
  - Influences results to be positive
  - Pygmalion unique to *investigator driving positive benefit*
- Hawthorne Effect
  - Subjects/investigators behave differently because of study

Lead Time Bias

- Screening test identifies disease earlier
- Makes survival appear longer when it is not
- Consider:
  - Avg. time from detection of breast lump to death = 5 years
  - Screening test identifies cancer earlier
  - Time from detection to death = 7 years

Recall Bias

- Inaccurate recall of past events by study subjects
- Common in survey studies
- Consider:
  - Patients with disabled children are asked about lifestyle during pregnancy many years ago

Procedure Bias

- Occurs when one group receives procedure (e.g., surgery) and another no procedure
- More care/attention given to procedure patients

Late-look Bias

- Patients with severe disease do not get studied because they die
- Example: Analysis of HIV+ patients shows the disease is asymptomatic

Observer Bias

- Investigators know exposure status of patient
- Examples:
  - Cardiologists interpret EKGs knowing patients have CAD
  - Pathologists review specimens knowing patients have cancer
- Avoided by blinding

Measurement Bias

- Sloppy research technique
- Blood pressure measured incorrectly in one arm
- Protocol not followed

Ways to Reduce Bias

- Randomization
  - Limits confounding and selection bias
- Matching of groups
- Blinding
- Crossover studies

Crossover Study

- Subjects randomly assigned to a sequence of treatments
- Group A: Placebo 8 weeks –> Drug 8 Weeks
- Group B: Drug 8 weeks –> Placebo 8 weeks
- Subjects serve as their own control
  - Avoids confounding (same subject!)
- Drawback is that effect can "carry over"
- Avoid by having a "wash out" period

Crossover Study

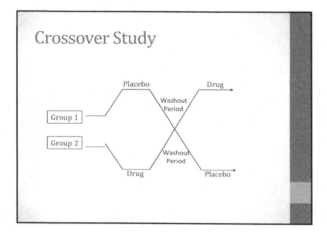

Effect Modification

- Not a type of bias (point of confusion)
- Occurs when 3rd factor alters effect
- Consider:
  - Drug A is shown to increase risk of DVT
  - To cause DVT, Drug A *requires* Gene X
  - Gene X is an effect modifier

Effect Modification

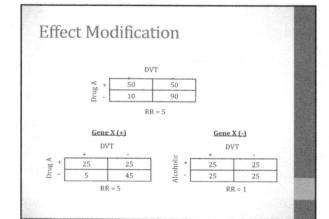

Effect Mod. vs. Confounding

- Confounding:
  - A 3rd variable *distorts* effect on outcome
  - Smoking and alcohol
  - Alcohol appears associated with cancer (positive)
  - Real effect of exposure on outcome distorted by confounder
- Effect modification:
  - A 3rd variable *maintains* effect but only in one group
  - There is a real effect of exposure on outcome
  - Effect requires presence of 3rd variable

Effect Mod. vs. Confounding
Example

- People who take drug A appear to have increased rates of lung cancer compared to people who do not take drug A
- Drug A is taken only by smokers
- If we break down data into smokers and non-smokers, there will be NO relationship between Drug A and cancer
- Smoking is the real cause
- Drug A has no effect
- This is confounding

Effect Mod. vs. Confounding
Example

- People who take drug A appear to have increased rates of lung cancer compared to people who do not take drug A
- Drug A activates gene X to cause cancer
- If we break down data into gene X (+) and (-), there will be a relationship between Drug A and cancer but only in gene X (+)
- Drug A *does* have effect (different from confounding)
- But drug A requires another factor (gene X)
- This is effect modification (not a form of bias)

Latent Period

- Occurs when diseases take a long time
- Studies of exposure/drugs shorter than this period will show no effect
- Consider:
  - Aspirin given to prevent heart attack
  - Patients studied for one month
  - No benefit seen
  - This is due to latency: atherosclerosis takes years to progress
  - Need to study for longer

Summary

Biases ———— Attrition
Selection ——— Sampling
Confounding ——— Berkson's
Hawthorne Effect
Pygmalion Effect
Lead Time
Recall
Procedure
Late-look
Observer
Measurement

Effect Modification
Latent Period

Clinical Trials

Jason Ryan, MD, MPH

Clinical Trials

- Experimental studies with human subjects
- Aim: determine benefit of therapy
  - Drug, surgery, etc.

Clinical Trials

- Suppose we want to know if drug X saves lives
- Obvious test:
  - Give drug X to some patients
  - See how long they live (or how many die)

Clinical Trials

- Several problems
  - Maybe survival (or death) same with no drug X
  - Group with drug KNOWS they are getting drug
  - Investigators KNOW patients getting drug
  - Behavior may change based on knowledge of drug

Clinical Trial Features

- Control
- Randomization
- Blinding

Control

- One group receives therapy
- Other group no therapy (control group)
- Ensures changes in therapy group not due to chance